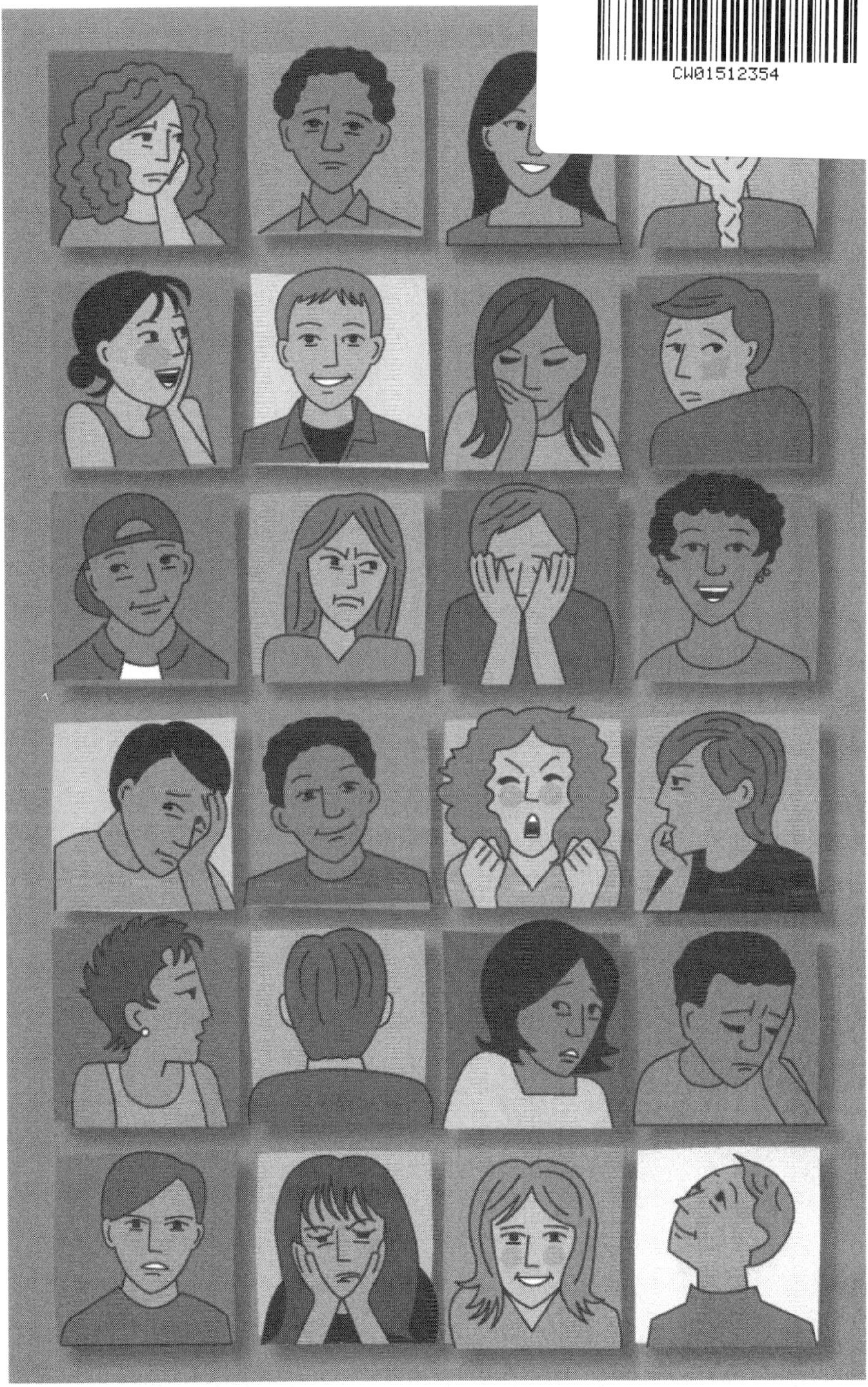

This booklet is for you

If your mom, dad, or an adult close to you has cancer, this booklet is for you.

Here you can read about what has helped other teens get through this tough time.

Doctors, nurses, social workers, friends, and family are working hard to help your mom or dad get better. You are a very important part of that team, too.

In the weeks and months ahead, you may feel a whole range of emotions. Some days will be good, and things might seem like they used to. Other days may be harder.

This booklet can help prepare you for some of the things you might face. It can also help you learn to handle living with a parent or relative who has cancer.

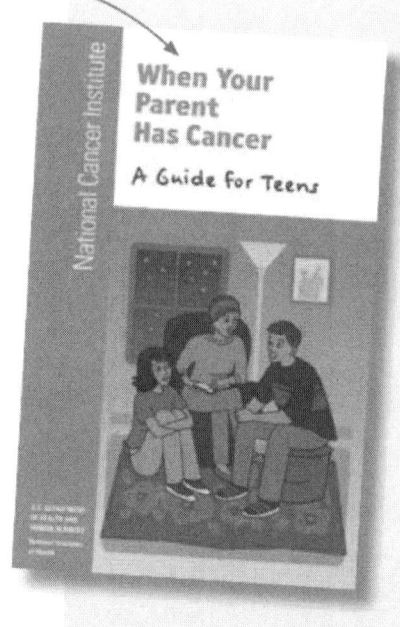

National Cancer Institute

When Your Parent Has Cancer

A Guide for Teens

Get free copies of this booklet from our Web site:

www.cancer.gov/publications

or by calling NCI's Cancer Information Service at 1-800-4-CANCER (1-800-422-6237).

Acknowledgments

We would like to thank the many teens, health care providers, and scientists who helped to develop and review this booklet.

How to use this booklet

You may want to read this booklet cover to cover. Or maybe you'll just read those sections that interest you most. Some teens pull the booklet out now and again when they need it.

You may want to share this booklet with your mom, dad, brothers, and sisters. It might help you bring up something that has been on your mind. You could ask people in your family to read a certain chapter and then talk about it together later.

We've put words that may be new to you in **bold**. Turn to the glossary at the back of this booklet for their definitions.

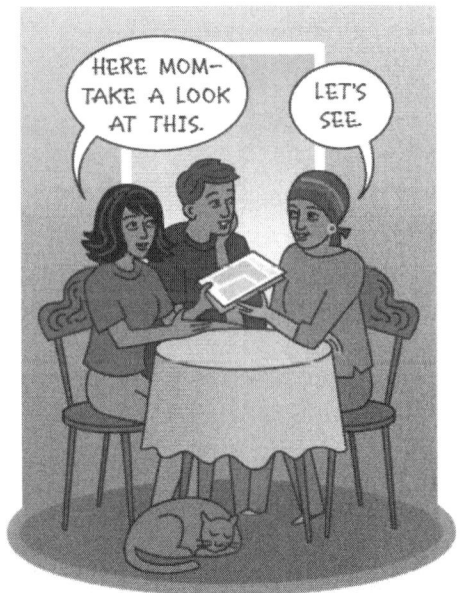

Wherever you go,

    go with all your heart.

               —Confucius

Table of contents

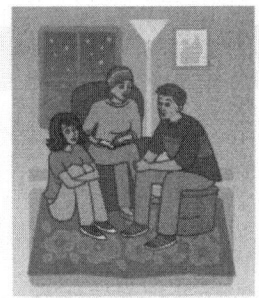

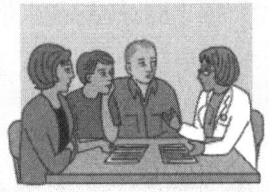

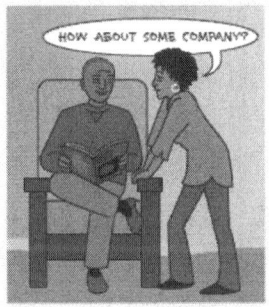

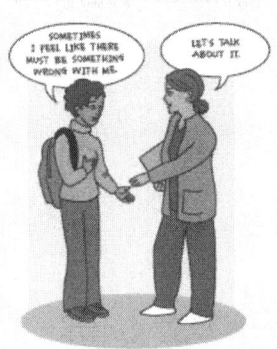

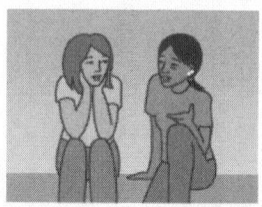

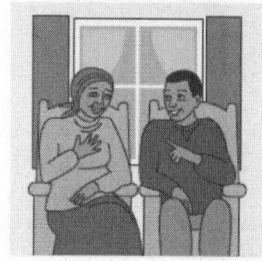

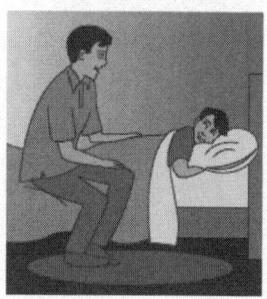

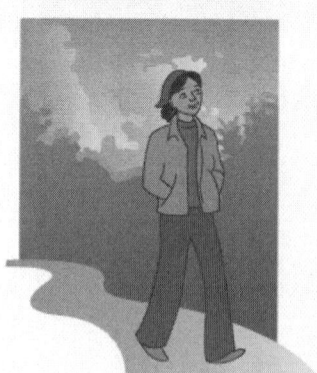

Chapter 1

You've just learned that your parent has cancer

You've just learned that one of the most important people in your life has **cancer**. Do you feel shocked, numb, angry, or afraid? Do you feel like life is unfair? One thing is certain—you don't feel good.

"I knew something was wrong the minute I walked in the kitchen. My mom was so quiet. Then Mom told me she has cancer. I felt like I was going to faint. I could barely hold the tears back. I felt so scared. I ran to my room and just sat on the bed for the longest time. I called my best friend and kind of lost it. —Sarah, age 16

For now, try to focus on these facts:

➡ **Many people survive cancer.** There are about 12 million cancer survivors living in the U.S. today. That's because scientists are discovering new and better ways to find and treat cancer. During this really tough time, it will help you to have hope.

➡ **You're not alone.** Right now it might seem that no one else in the world feels the way you do. In a way you're right. No one can feel exactly like you do. But it might help to know that many teens have a parent who has cancer. Talking to others may help you sort out your feelings. Remember, you are not alone.

➡ **You're not to blame.** Cancer is a disease with various causes, many of which doctors don't fully understand. None of these causes has anything to do with what you've done, thought, or said.

➡ **Balance is important.** Many teens feel like their parent's cancer is always on their mind. Others try to avoid it. Try to strike a balance. You can be concerned about your parent and still stay connected with people and activities that you care about.

➡ **Knowledge is power.** It can help to learn more about cancer and cancer treatments. Sometimes what you imagine is actually worse than the reality.

"I used to be a real easygoing, happy person. Since my dad got cancer I started blowing up over little things. My counselor at school got me in a group of kids who have a mom or dad with cancer. Meeting with kids who are going through the same thing helps a lot."
—Aaron, age 14

Your feelings

As you deal with your parent's cancer, you'll probably feel all kinds of things. Many other teens who have a parent with cancer have felt the same way you do now. Some of these emotions are listed below. Think about people you can talk with about your feelings.

Check off the feelings you have:

scared

☐ My world is falling apart.

☐ I'm afraid that my parent might die.

☐ I'm afraid that someone else in my family might catch cancer. (They can't.)

☐ I'm afraid that something might happen to my parent at home, and I won't know what to do.

It's normal to feel scared when your parent has cancer. Some of your fears may be real. Others may be based on things that won't happen. And some fears may lessen over time.

guilty

☐ I feel guilty because I'm healthy and my parent is sick.

☐ I feel guilty when I laugh and have fun.

You may feel bad about having fun when your parent is sick. However, having fun doesn't mean that you care any less. In fact, it will probably help your parent to see you doing things you enjoy.

angry

- [ ] I am mad that my mom or dad got sick.
- [ ] I am upset at the doctors.
- [ ] I am angry at God for letting this happen.
- [ ] I am angry at myself for feeling the way I do.

Anger often covers up other feelings that are harder to show. Try not to let your anger build up.

neglected

- [ ] I feel left out.
- [ ] I don't get any attention.
- [ ] No one ever tells me what's going on.
- [ ] My family never talks anymore.

When a parent has cancer, it's common for the family's focus to change. Some people in the family may feel left out. Your parent with cancer may be using his or her energy to get better. Your well parent may be focused on helping your parent with cancer. Your parents don't mean for you to feel left out. It just happens because so much is going on.

When you come to the end of your rope,

☐ No one understands what I'm going through.

☐ My friends don't come over anymore.

☐ My friends don't seem to know what to say to me anymore.

We look at some things you can do to help situations with friends in Chapter 8. For now, try to remember that these feelings won't last forever.

☐ I'm sometimes embarrassed to be out in public with my sick parent.

☐ I don't know how to answer people's questions.

Many teens who feel embarrassed about having a parent with cancer say it gets easier to deal with over time.

What you're feeling is normal

There is no one "right" way to feel. And you're not alone—many other teens in your situation have felt the same way. Some have said that having a parent with cancer changes the way they look at things in life. Some even said that it made them stronger.

tie a knot and hang on. —Franklin D. Roosevelt

Dealing with your feelings

A lot of people are uncomfortable sharing their feelings. They ignore them and hope they'll go away. Other people choose to act cheerful when they're really not. They think that by acting upbeat they won't feel sad or angry anymore. This may help for a little while, but not over the long run. Actually, holding your feelings inside can keep you from getting the help you need.

Try these tips:

➡ Talk with family and friends who you feel close to. You owe it to yourself.

➡ Write down your thoughts in a journal.

➡ Join a **support group** to talk with other teens who are facing some of the same things you are. Or meet with a counselor. We'll learn more about these ideas in Chapter 7.

It is probably hard to imagine right now, but, if you let yourself, you can grow stronger as a person through this experience.

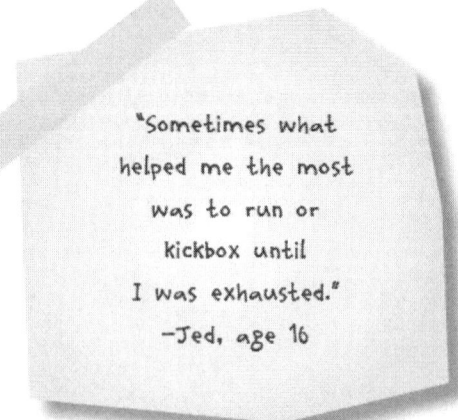

"Sometimes what helped me the most was to run or kickbox until I was exhausted."
—Jed, age 16

Many kids think that they need to protect their parents by not making them worry. They think that they have to be perfect and not cause any trouble because one of their parents is sick. If you feel this way, remember that no one can be perfect all the time. You need time to vent, to feel sad, and to be happy. Try to let your parents know how you feel—even if you have to start the conversation.

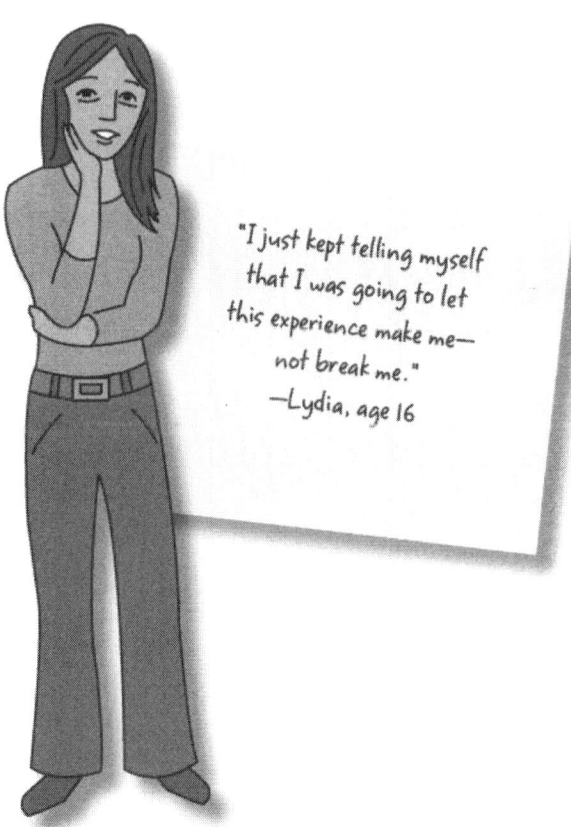

"I just kept telling myself that I was going to let this experience make me— not break me."
—Lydia, age 16

"After Dad got cancer, my big sister always seemed to be making excuses to get out of the house. One day, I just told her off. Instead of getting mad, she started crying. She said she couldn't stand seeing Dad hurting. I told her I felt the same way. Now we talk more and keep each other going. It's good." —Jamie, age 13

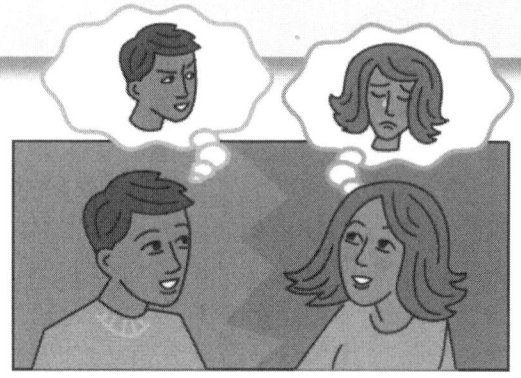

Experience is what you get
by not having it
when you need it.
—Anonymous

Chapter 2

Learning about cancer

Learning about cancer will help you understand what your parent is going through. Knowing more about cancer and how it's treated can take some of the fear away. Some of what you have seen or heard about cancer may not apply to your parent. Most people feel better when they know what to expect.

"When Dad told me he had cancer, I got really scared. Everything I'd always heard about cancer was just terrible. Then I thought, 'Hey, what do I really know about cancer?' The answer was, 'Not much.' So I started reading books and stuff on the Internet. My dad even told me that some of what I found on the Web wasn't right for the kind of cancer he has. Cancer is still pretty scary, but I've learned that people survive it. I'm not so afraid anymore." —Abdul, age 14

Here are a few things to remember:

➡ Nothing you did, thought, or said caused your parent to get cancer.

➡ You can't catch cancer from another person.

➡ Scientists are discovering new and better ways to find and treat cancer.

➡ Many people survive cancer.

9

What is cancer?

Doctors have found more than 100 different types of cancer. Cancer is a group of many related diseases that begin in **cells**, the body's basic unit of life. To understand cancer, it's helpful to know what happens when normal cells become cancer cells.

Normally, cells grow and divide to make more cells only when the body needs them. This orderly process helps keep the body healthy. Sometimes, however, cells keep dividing when new cells aren't needed. These extra cells form a mass of **tissue** called a growth, or **tumor**. Tumors can be **benign** or **malignant**. Some cancers do not form a tumor. For example, **leukemia** is a cancer of the **bone marrow** and blood.

➡ **Benign tumors aren't cancer.** They can often be removed and don't spread to other parts of the body.

➡ **Malignant tumors are cancer.** Cells in these tumors are abnormal and divide and grow without control or order. They can invade and damage nearby tissues and also spread to organs in other parts of the body. The spread of cancer from one part of the body to another is called **metastasis**.

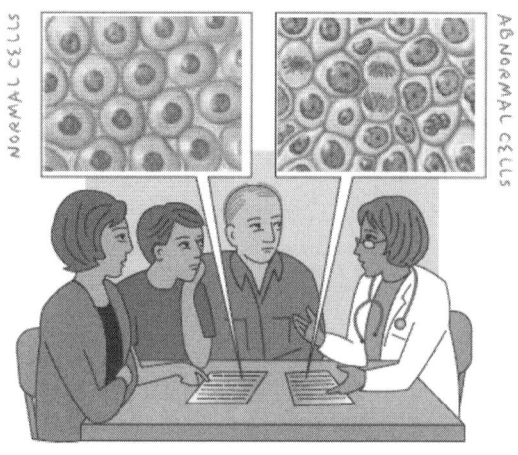

Most cancers are named for the organ or type of cell in which they begin. For example, cancer that begins in the lung is called **lung cancer**.

Why do people get cancer?

The causes of most cancers are not known. Scientists are still learning about things that may put people at a higher risk for certain types of cancer. **Risk factors** for cancer include age, a **family history** of certain cancers, use of tobacco products, being exposed to radiation or certain chemicals, infection with certain viruses or bacteria, and certain genetic changes.

Although no one can tell the future, it is good to keep in mind that most cancers are not passed down from parent to child. That is, they are not **inherited**. However, a family history of cancer can sometimes be a risk factor. It may help to talk with your parent or a doctor to learn more about the kind of cancer that your parent has.

Can doctors cure cancer?

Every year scientists discover better ways to treat cancer. That means many people are successfully treated for cancer. However, doctors are careful not to use the word "cure" until a patient remains free of cancer for several years. Cancer treatment may cause a **remission**, which means that the doctor can't find signs of cancer. But sometimes the cancer comes back. This is called a **relapse** or **recurrence**. Whether your parent can be cured of cancer depends on many things, and no booklet can tell you exactly what to expect. It is best to talk with your parent and his or her doctor or nurse.

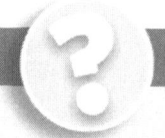

To learn more and get answers to your questions, you can contact NCI through its:

- **Web site:** www.cancer.gov

- **Phone:** 1-800-4-CANCER (1-800-422-6237)
  Monday through Friday, 8:00 a.m. to 8:00 p.m. Eastern Time

- **Online Chat:** www.cancer.gov/livehelp
  Monday through Friday, 8:00 a.m. to 11:00 p.m. Eastern Time

- **E-mail:** cancergovstaff@mail.nih.gov

All of our services are free and confidential.

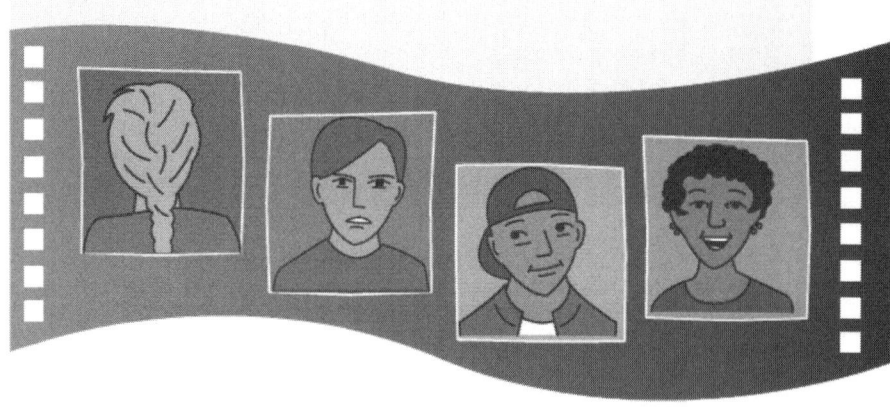

Courage is the first of human qualities
because it is the quality which
guarantees the others.

—Aristotle

Chapter 3

Cancer treatment

Many teens want to know what to expect during their parent's cancer treatment. This chapter briefly explains different treatments, how they work, and their **side effects**. You will probably have more questions after reading this chapter. It may help to talk with your parents or ask if you can talk with a nurse or social worker.

"Seeing my dad in pain was the worst. One day I just told him how bad I felt for him. He said that he actually looked a lot worse than he felt. I know he's having a hard time, but knowing he doesn't hurt as much as I thought he did made me feel a lot better."
  Ashley, age 15

How does treatment work?

Cancer treatment aims to destroy cancer cells or stop them from growing. The type of treatment your parent will be given depends on:

→ The type of cancer

→ Whether the cancer has spread

→ Your parent's age and general health

→ Your parent's medical history

→ Whether the cancer is newly **diagnosed** or is a recurrence

Remember that there are more than 100 different types of cancer. Each type is treated differently. For information about the people who will be treating your parent, see Chart A in the back of this booklet.

13

What are treatment side effects?

Cancer treatments destroy cancer cells, but they may also harm healthy tissues or organs in the process. This harm, or problem, is called a side effect. Some side effects, like feeling sick to the stomach, go away shortly after treatment, but others, like feeling tired, may last for a while after treatment has ended. Some people have few side effects from cancer treatment, while others have more.

Side effects vary from person to person, even among people who are receiving the same treatment. Your parent's doctor will explain what side effects your parent may have, and how to manage them.

Write down what treatment your mom or dad will get:

_____

_____

_____

_____

_____

_____

_____

_____

Use the chart on the next two pages to find out more about different types of cancer treatment.

TREATMENT CHART

This chart describes six types of cancer treatment, how they're done, and some side effects. Your parent may get one or more of these treatments. Depending on the exact treatment, he or she may visit the doctor during the day, or stay overnight in the hospital.

Treatment	What is it?	How is it done?	What may happen as a result? (side effects)
Surgery Also called an operation	The removal of a solid tumor	A surgeon operates to remove the tumor. Drugs are used so that the patient is asleep during surgery.	• Pain after the surgery • Feeling tired • Other side effects depend on the area of the body and the extent of the operation
Radiation therapy Also called radiotherapy	The use of high-energy rays or high-energy particles to kill cancer cells and shrink tumors	Radiation may come from a machine outside the body or from radioactive material placed in the body near the cancer cells.	• Feeling tired • Red or sore skin • Other side effects depend on the area of the body and the dose of radiation
Chemotherapy Also called chemo	The use of medicine to destroy cancer cells	The medicine can be given as a pill, as an injection (shot), or through an **intravenous (IV)** line. It is often given in cycles that alternate between treatment and rest periods.	• Feeling sick to the stomach or throwing up • Diarrhea or constipation • Hair loss • Feeling very tired • Mouth sores

Treatment chart continues on next page.

TREATMENT CHART (continued from previous page)			
Treatment	What is it?	How is it done?	What may happen as a result? (side effects)
Stem cell transplantation Can be a bone marrow transplantation (BMT) or a peripheral blood stem cell transplantation (PBSCT)	The use of **stem cells** found in either the bone marrow or the blood. This repairs stem cells that were destroyed by high doses of chemo and/or radiation therapy.	Stem cell transplantation uses stem cells from the patient or from donors. In many cases the donors are family members. The patient gets these stem cells through an IV line.	The side effects can be much like those from chemo and radiation therapy. In some cases, the side effects may be more serious.
Hormone therapy	A treatment that adds, blocks, or removes **hormones**. Hormone therapy is used to slow or stop the growth of some types of cancer.	Hormone therapy can be given as a pill, as an injection, or through a patch worn on the skin. Sometimes surgery is needed to remove the glands that make specific hormones.	• Feeling hot • Feeling tired • Weight changes • Mood changes
Biological therapy Also called immunotherapy	Biological therapy uses the body's own defense system (the **immune system**) to fight cancer.	Patients may be given medicine in pills, as an injection, or through an IV line.	Flu-like symptoms such as: • Chills • Fever • Muscle aches • Weakness • Feeling sick to the stomach or throwing up • Diarrhea

In addition to getting one or more cancer treatments, your parent will also get tests to find out how well the cancer is responding to treatment. A list of common tests can be found in Chart B in the back of this booklet.

Things to look for

Some treatments may make your parent more likely to get an infection. This happens because cancer treatment can affect the white blood cells, which are the cells that fight infection. An infection can make your mom or dad sicker. So your parent may need to stay away from crowded places or people who have an illness that he or she could catch (such as a cold, the flu, or chicken pox).

You may need to:

➡ Wash your hands often with soap and water, or use a hand sanitizer, to keep from spreading germs.

➡ Avoid bringing home friends who are sick or have a cold.

➡ Stay away from your parent if you are sick or have a fever.

Talk with your parent if you aren't sure what to do.

The waiting

It's hard to wait to see whether the treatment will work. Your parent's doctor may try one treatment, then another. One day your parent may feel a lot better. The next day or week he or she may feel sick again. Treatment can go on for months or sometimes years. This emotional roller coaster is hard on everyone.

Who can answer my other questions?

Ask your parent or other trusted adults any questions that you have. Ask your dad or mom if it is okay to go with them to their appointment.

Perhaps your parent can arrange for you to talk with their doctor, nurse, or social worker to learn more. It will help to bring a list of questions with you.

When you talk with them, don't hesitate to:

➡ Ask what new words mean. Ask for information to be explained in another way, if what the doctor says is confusing.

➡ Ask to see a model or a picture of what the doctor is talking about. Ask what videos or podcasts you can watch to learn more.

➡ Ask about support groups for young people that meet online or in your community.

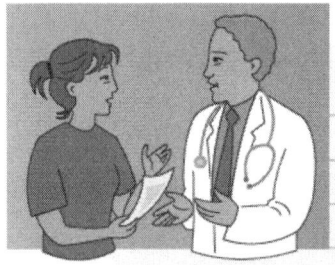

"I had questions but didn't know who to talk to. I asked my mom if I could go with her to her doctor's visit, and she said yes. The first time I just sat there. The next time the doctor asked if I had questions—so I asked a couple. It was easier than I thought it would be." —Katie, age 14

Questions you might want to ask

- What kind of cancer does my parent have?
- Will my parent get better?
- Does this kind of cancer run in families?

Questions about the treatment

- What kind of treatment will my parent get? Will my parent get more than one type of treatment?
- How does the treatment work?
- How do people feel when they get this treatment? Does it hurt?
- How often is this treatment given? How long will treatment take?
- Does the treatment change how people look, feel, or act?
- What if this treatment doesn't work?
- Where is the treatment given? Can I go along?

Here's space to write down your own questions:

_____

_____

_____

_____

_____

▶ It's okay to ask these questions more than once.

19

Want to visit?

If your parent is in the hospital, you may be nervous about visiting. Learn ahead of time how your parent is doing and what to expect. Remember that they are still the same person, even though they are sick. Don't be afraid to ask your parent questions and share your thoughts. You can also call, write, and e-mail them.

"I really wanted to visit, but the hospital made me nervous. I wasn't crazy about the smell and didn't like seeing Dad hooked up to machines. I made excuses not to visit, but I missed him too much. Then one day a neighbor drove me over to the hospital after school. I took my homework and did some of it there. Dad looked happy just watching me—and that made me forget about how strange it was to be in this place." —Keisha, age 13

Where to go for more information

To learn more about the type of cancer your mom or dad has, visit our site (**www.cancer.gov**). You can also call our Cancer Information Service at 1-800-4-CANCER (1-800-422-6237) to talk with an information specialist. All calls are free and confidential.

Chapter 4

What your parent may be feeling

Knowing what your parent may be feeling could help you figure out how to help, or at least to understand where he or she is coming from. You may be surprised to learn that they are feeling a lot of the same things you are:

➡ **Sad or depressed.** People with cancer sometimes can't do things they used to do. They may miss these activities and their friends. Feeling sad or down can range from a mild case of the blues to **depression**, which a doctor can treat.

➡ **Afraid.** Your parent may be afraid of how cancer will change his or her life and the lives of family members. He or she may be scared about treatment. Your parent may even be scared that he or she will die.

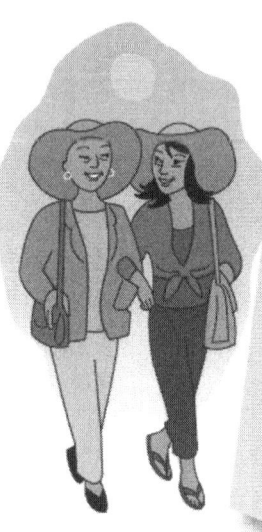

"My mom lost all her hair after chemo. She started wearing hats. People stared at us. I felt really bad that I was embarrassed to be with her. Then my mom just came out and asked me what I was thinking. When I told her, she said she wasn't crazy about the new bald look either, but that she was glad to be alive. Now I see my mom first as one very brave woman. I don't care who stares."
—Ming, age 16

➡️ **Anxious.** Your parent may be worried about a lot of things. Your mom or dad may feel stressed about going to work or paying the bills. Or he or she may be concerned about looking different because of treatment. And your mom or dad is probably very concerned about how you are doing. All these worries may upset your parent.

➡️ **Angry.** Cancer treatment and its side effects can be difficult to go through. Anger sometimes comes from feelings that are hard to show, such as fear or frustration. Chances are your parent is angry at the disease, not at you.

➡️ **Lonely.** People with cancer often feel lonely or distant from others. They may find that their friends have a hard time dealing with their cancer and may not visit. They may be too sick to take part in activities they used to enjoy. They may feel that no one understands what they're going through.

➡️ **Hopeful.** There are many reasons for your parent to feel hopeful. Millions of people who have had cancer are alive today. People with cancer can lead active lives, even during treatment. Your parent's chances of surviving cancer are better today than ever before.

All these feelings are normal for people living with cancer. You might want to share this list with your mom or dad.

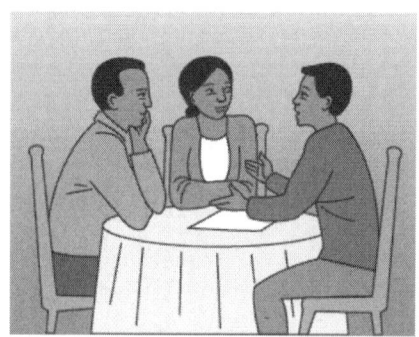

Do what you can, with what you have,

Chapter 5

Changes in your family

Changing routines and responsibilities

Whatever your family situation, chances are that things have changed since your parent got sick. This chapter looks at some of these changes and ways that other teens have dealt with them.

Does this sound like your home?

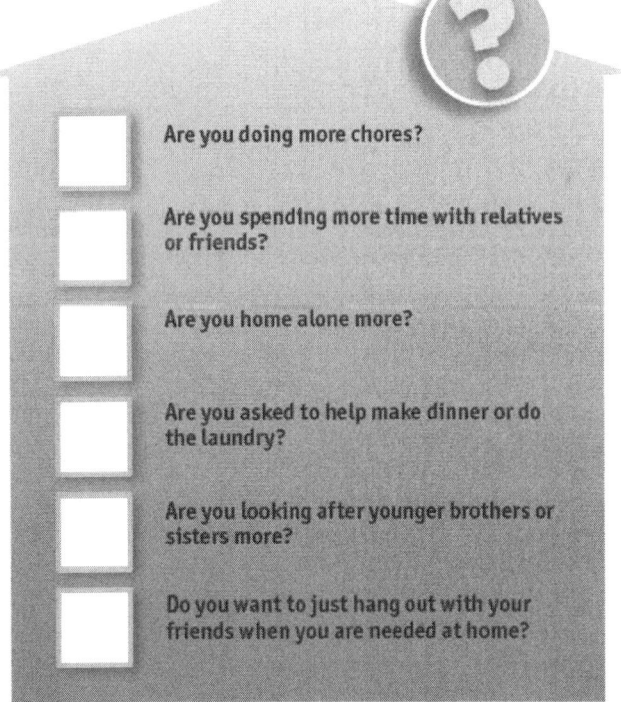

Are you doing more chores?

Are you spending more time with relatives or friends?

Are you home alone more?

Are you asked to help make dinner or do the laundry?

Are you looking after younger brothers or sisters more?

Do you want to just hang out with your friends when you are needed at home?

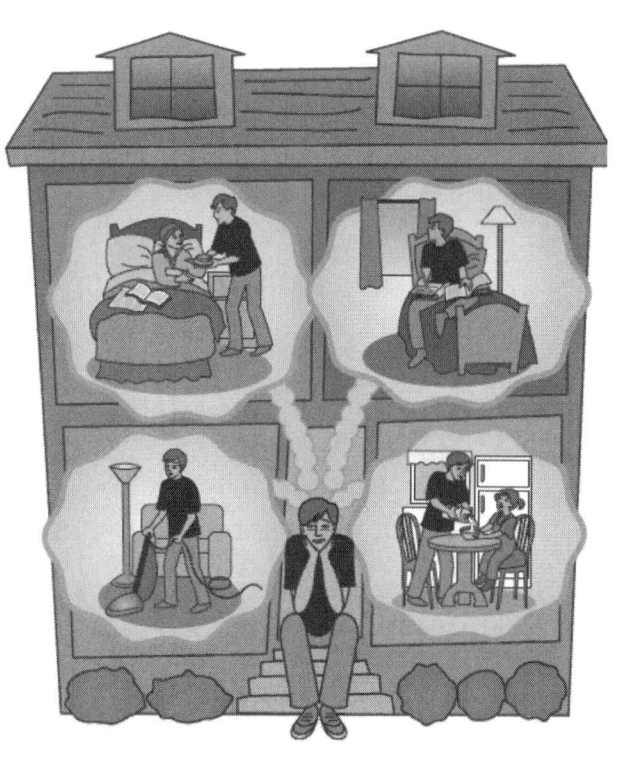

Let your parents know if you feel that there is more to do than you can handle. Together, you can work it out.

"After Mom got cancer, I got mad at everything. It wasn't fair that I had to watch my little brother and clean. I felt like I was going to lose it, but tried to stay cool and told my mom how hard things were. Now I still have chores, but my little brother goes to a friend's after school, so that I can go to soccer. My mom's awesome. She really understood." —Brandon, age 15

Touching base when things are changing

Families say that it helps to make time to talk together, even if it's only for a short time each week. Talking can help your family stay connected.

Here are some things to consider when talking with:

Brothers and sisters

➡ If you are the oldest child, your brothers or sisters may look to you for support. Help them as much as you can. It's okay to let them know that you're having a tough time, too.

➡ If you are looking to your older brother or sister for help, tell them how you are feeling. They can help, but won't have all the answers.

"I'm doing the best job I can."

"How can we work together to get through this?"

Try saying something like this...

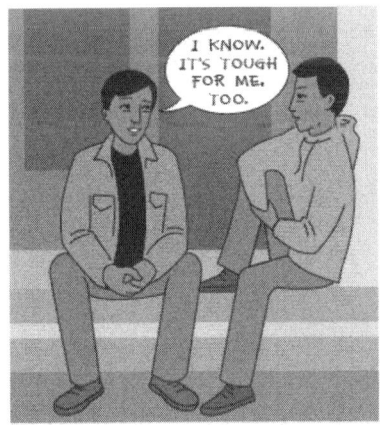

I KNOW. IT'S TOUGH FOR ME. TOO.

I am only one,
but I am one.
I cannot do
everything,
but I can do
something.
—Edward Everett Hale

Your parent who is well

- Expect your parent to feel some stress, just as you do.

- Your parent may snap at you. He or she may not always do or say the right thing.

- Lend a hand when you can.

Try saying something like this...

"How are you doing?"

"Is there anything I can do to help you out?"

Your parent with cancer

- Your mom or dad may be sick from the treatment or just very tired. Or maybe your parent will feel okay and want your company.

- Try talking if your mom or dad feels up to it. Let your parent know how much you love them.

Try saying something like this...

"I love you."

"Can I get you anything?"

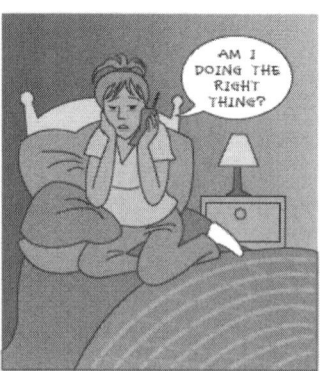

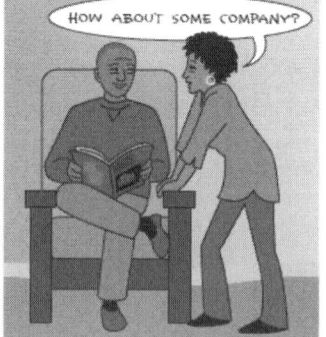

Keeping family and friends in the loop ◀

Is it getting to be too much to answer the phone and tell people how your mom or dad is doing? That can be a lot for anyone. Ask others to help you share news of how your parent is doing and what help your family needs. Maybe a relative or family friend can be the contact person. Some families use telephone chains. Others use e-mail, a blog, or a social media site.

Growing stronger as a family

Some families can grow apart for a while when a parent has cancer. But there are ways to help your family grow stronger and closer. Teens who saw their families grow closer say that it happened because people in their family:

"I always took my parents' attention for granted. But after Dad got sick, nobody paid much attention to me. I know everybody has a lot to worry about, but it really hurt. Finally, I wrote a note to them. And they understood! I feel closer to my parents now." —Lisa, age 15

➡ **Tried** to put themselves in the other person's shoes and thought about how they would feel if they were the other person.

➡ **Understood** that even though people reacted differently to situations, they were all hurting. Some cried a lot. Others showed little emotion. Some used humor to get by.

➡ **Learned** to respect and talk about differences. The more they asked about how others were feeling, the more they could help each other.

Asking others for help

You and your family may need support from others. It can be hard to ask. Yet most of the time people really want to help you and your family.

People who your mom, dad, or you may ask for help:

Aunts, uncles, and grandparents

Family friends

Neighbors

Teachers or coaches

School nurses or guidance counselors

People from your religious community

Your friends or their parents

(Add your own) _____

Things people can do to help:

Go grocery shopping or run errands

Make meals

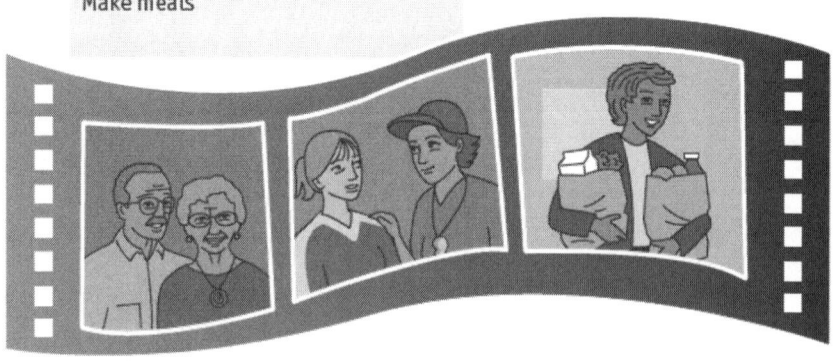

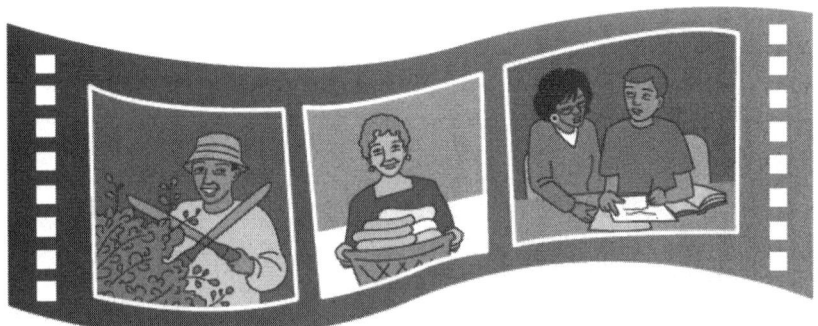

Mow the lawn

Do chores around the house

Keep your parent company

(Add your own) _____

Other ways people can help you and your family:

Give rides to school, practice, or appointments

Help with homework

Invite you over for a meal or a day trip

Talk with and listen to you

(Add your own) _____

Your relationship with your parents ◀······

Your mom or dad may ask you to take on more responsibility than other kids your age. You might resent it at first. Then again, you may learn a lot from the experience and grow to appreciate the trust your parents have in you. See Chapter 7 for tips on talking with your parents.

"I never used to get sick before Mom got cancer. But then I started getting headaches. My stomach hurt all the time, too. I started wondering if something was wrong with me. I talked to a nurse, and she said that stress can cause a lot of that stuff. She gave me some great advice and said I could talk with her whenever I wanted to. Slowly, I'm feeling better."

Kira, age 15

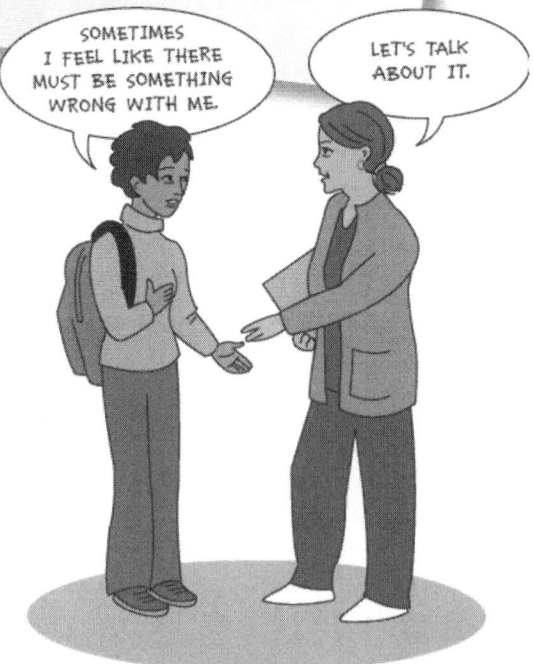

Chapter 6

Taking care of yourself

It's important to "stay fit"—both inside and out. This chapter offers tips to help you keep on track during this experience.

Dealing with stress

Stress can make you forgetful, frustrated, and more likely to catch a cold or the flu. Here are some tips that have helped other teens manage stress. Check one or two things to do each week.

Take care of your mind and body

Stay connected.

☐ Spend some time at a friend's house.

☐ Stay involved with sports or clubs.

Relax and get enough sleep.

☐ Take breaks. You'll have more energy and be in a better frame of mind.

☐ Get at least 8 hours of sleep each night.

☐ Pray or meditate.

☐ Make or listen to music.

Help others.

☐ Join a walk against cancer.

☐ Plan a bake sale or other charity event to raise money to fight cancer.

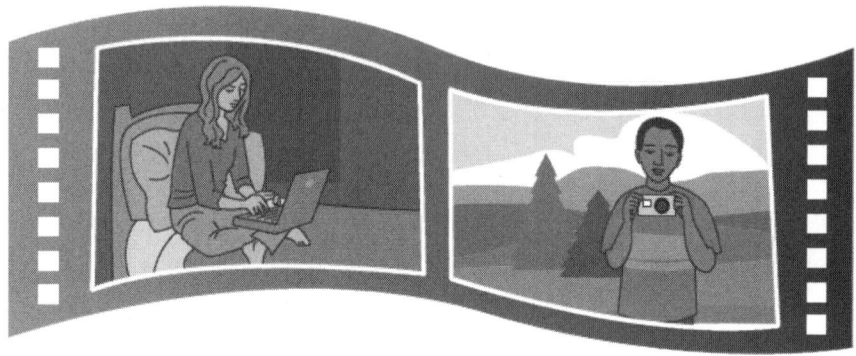

Avoid risky behaviors.

☐ Stay away from smoking, drinking, and taking drugs.

Put your creative side to work.

☐ Keep a journal to write down your thoughts and experiences.

☐ Draw, paint, or take photographs.

☐ Read biographies to learn what helped others make it through challenging times.

Eat and drink well.

☐ Drink plenty of water each day.

☐ In the evening, switch to caffeine-free drinks that won't keep you awake.

☐ Grab fresh fruit, whole-grain breads, and lean meats like chicken or turkey when you have a choice.

☐ Avoid sugary foods.

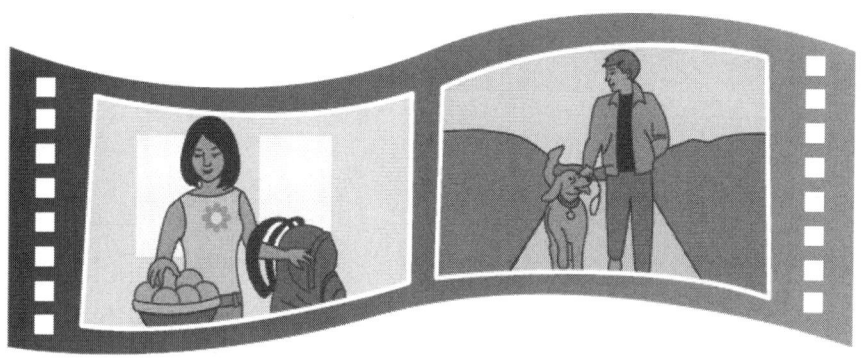

Be active.

- ☐ Play a sport, or go for a walk or run.
- ☐ Learn about different stretching and breathing exercises.

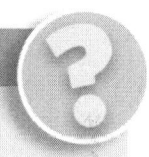

Did you know?

Exercise has been proven to make you feel better. Running, swimming, or even walking can help improve your mood.

The best thing about the future

is that it comes

only one day

at a time.

—Abraham Lincoln

Take steps to keep things simple

Staying organized can also keep your stress level under control. Here are some tips to get you started.

At home

- ☐ Make a list of things you want to do and put the most important ones at the top.
- ☐ Make a big calendar to help your family stay on top of things.

At school

- ☐ Try to get as much done in school as you can.
- ☐ Let your teachers know what's happening at home, without using it as an excuse.
- ☐ Talk to your teachers or a counselor if you are falling behind.

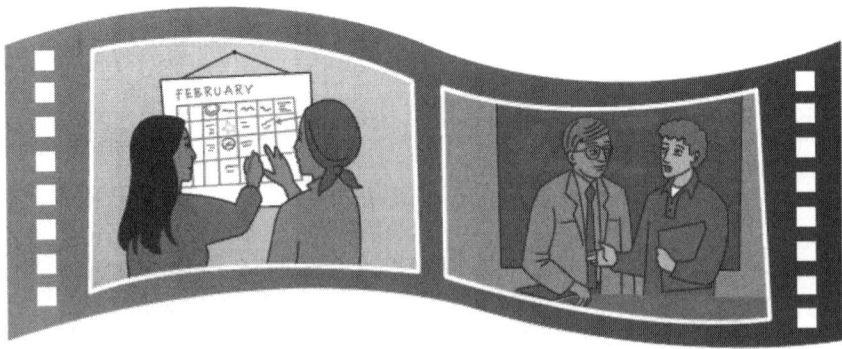

Get help when you feel down and out.

Many teens feel low or down when their parent is sick. It's normal to feel sad or "blue" during difficult times. However, if these feelings last for 2 weeks or more and start to interfere with things you used to enjoy, you may be depressed. The good news is that there is hope and there is help. Often, talking with a counselor can help. Below are some signs that you may need to see a counselor.

➡ Are you:

- ☐ Feeling helpless and hopeless? Thinking that life has no meaning?
- ☐ Losing interest in being with family or friends?
- ☐ Finding that everything or everyone seems to get on your nerves?
- ☐ Feeling really angry a lot of the time?
- ☐ Thinking of hurting yourself?

➡ Do you find that you are:

- ☐ Losing interest in the activities you used to enjoy?
- ☐ Eating too little or a lot more than usual?
- ☐ Crying easily or many times each day?
- ☐ Using drugs or alcohol to help you forget?
- ☐ Sleeping more than you used to? Less than you used to?
- ☐ Feeling tired a lot?

If you answered "yes" to any of these questions, it's important to talk to someone you trust. Read more about seeing a counselor or joining a support group in Chapter 7.

35

"Things weren't easy between me and my dad. We fought about everything. After he got cancer, I felt really bad. Then the nurse told me about this support group. I ended up going with a friend. At first I just listened. Then I realized they were going through some of the same things that I was and actually had some helpful advice. Dad and I talk more now and even laugh about the dumb fights we had." —Alex, age 17

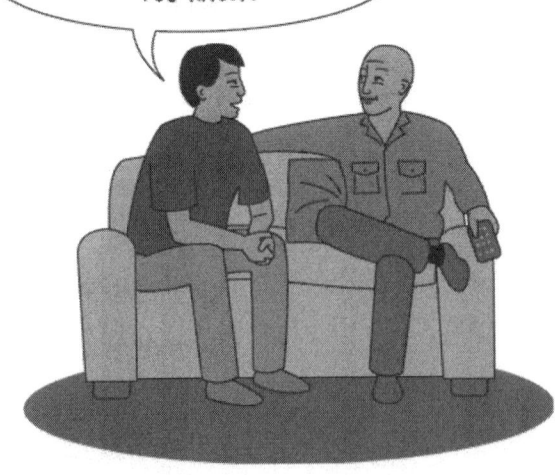

Chapter 7

Finding support

It may not be easy to reach out for support—but there are people who can help you. This chapter has tips to help you talk with your parent(s), reach out to a counselor, and/or join a support group. Read on to find out what's worked for other teens.

Tips for talking with your parent

Prepare before you talk.

Step 1: Think about what you want to say.

Step 2: Think about how your parent might react. How will you respond to him or her?

Find a good time and place.

Step 1: Ask your mom or dad if they have a few minutes to talk.

Step 2: Find a private place—maybe in your room or on the front steps. Or maybe you can talk while taking a walk, shooting hoops, or doing an activity you both enjoy.

Take things slowly.

Step 1: Don't expect to solve everything right away. Difficult problems often don't have simple solutions.

Step 2: Work together to find a way through these challenges. Some conversations will go better than others.

Keep it up.

Step 1: Don't think you have to have just one big conversation. Have lots of small ones.

Step 2: Make time to talk a little each day if you can, even if it's just for a few minutes.

Sometimes...
talking to friends
is not enough.
When you're having
a hard time,
it can be helpful to talk
with a counselor or
social worker.

▶ Talking with a counselor

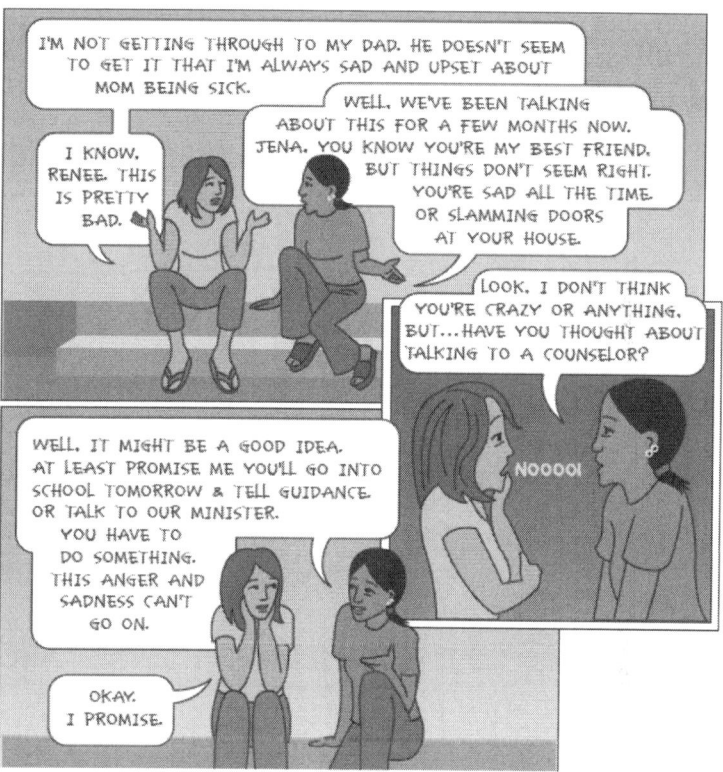

Jena listened to her best friend Renee and planned on talking with the counselor at her school. Other kids talk with social workers at the hospital. Going to a counselor doesn't mean you are crazy. It shows you have the courage to see that you need help to get through a very tough time.

Why go to a counselor?

Teens say it can be helpful to talk with someone outside the family—someone who doesn't take sides. A counselor is a person who will listen to you. They will help you find ways to better handle the things that bother you and gain strength in your situation.

Finding a counselor

➡ Talk with your mom, dad, or someone else you trust. Let them know you would like to talk to a counselor. Ask for help making appointments and getting to visits. Sometimes the counselor will even let you bring a friend.

➡ Ask a nurse or social worker at the hospital if they know someone you can talk to.

➡ Talk with your guidance counselor at school.

Don't be shy about asking for help.

You may think: "I can solve all my own problems." However, when faced with tough situations, both teens and adults need support from others!

Turn your face to the sun, and the shadows fall behind you. —Maori proverb

Joining a support group

Another good outlet is a support group. Some groups meet in person; others meet online. Some groups go out and have fun together. In these groups you'll meet other teens going through some of the same things that you are. At first this may not sound like something you want to do. Other teens say they thought the same thing—until they went to a meeting. They were surprised that so many others felt the same way they did and had advice that really seemed to work. A doctor, nurse, or social worker can help you find a support group.

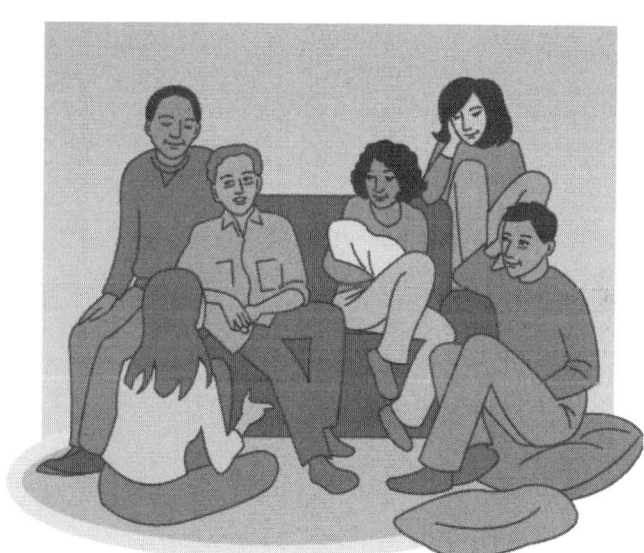

"Grandma raised me to care about school. But after she got cancer, I had too much on my mind. And there was a lot to do to take care of her when I got home from school. My grades started to slip. I told my guidance counselor what was going on, and she shared some things that had worked for others. Now, whenever things start to get me down, I talk with my guidance counselor, who helps me feel less stressed. What's best is that she keeps everything we talk about private."
—Nick, age 15

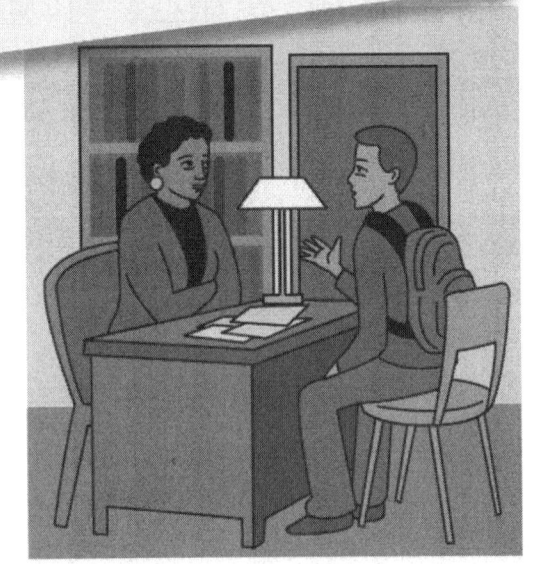

Chapter 8

You and your friends

Your friends are important to you, and you're important to them.

In the past, you could tell them everything. Now that your parent has cancer, it may seem like a lot is changing—even your friendships. Here are some things to think about:

Your friends may not know what to say.

→ It is hard for some people to know what to say. Others may think it's rude to ask questions.

→ Try to be gentle on friends who don't ask about your parent's cancer or how you are doing.

→ You may need to take the first step.

→ Try saying something like this...

"I still see my friends, but things are different now. A lot of what they talk about seems kind of lame. They are into going to school dances or to the mall. Sometimes I feel like an outsider. I worry a lot about my dad. Stuff like who won the basketball game just doesn't seem important now. Then I found out there was another kid at school whose dad has cancer. I have more in common with him than I do with friends I've known my whole life." Hamid, age 15

"Talking about what's going on with my mom/dad is hard. I know that it's not easy to ask questions. Is there anything you want to talk about or know?"

Your friends may ask tough questions.

→ You may not always feel like answering questions about your parent's cancer or treatment.

→ Try saying something like this: "talking about what's going on right now is hard, but it's nice of you to ask. The doctors are saying: [add in your own information here] . . ."

→ **If you don't feel like talking, try saying something like this...**

"Thanks for asking about my mom/dad, but would it be okay if we talked about this later?"

Your friends have their own lives.

→ It may feel like your friends don't care anymore. It might seem as though their lives are moving on, and yours isn't.

→ It can be hard to watch them get together with others or do things without you. But try to understand that they have their own lives, too. They aren't facing the situation you are right now, so it may be hard for them to relate.

→ **You might want to try saying something like this...**

"I miss hanging out together. I know that I've had a lot on my mind since my dad got sick. I'm glad we're still friends. Want to hang out tomorrow?"

44

Having fun and making new friends

Old friends

Even though you may have a lot on your mind, you can still get together with your friends and have a good time. If you can't leave home as much, ask if your friends can come over. Take time to relax. It's good for you. Make a list of fun things you and your friends like to do together. Then do them!

_____

_____

_____

_____

_____

_____

New friends

A lot is happening to you right now. Sometimes old friends move on. You may not have as much in common as you used to. The good news is that you may find yourself making new friends. Kids who used to just pass you in the halls may now ask you how you are doing. Kids who you used to be friends with may enter your life again. Be open to new friendships.

Going to support groups at the hospital or clinic is a good way to meet new friends. It helps to connect with people who are going through some of the same things that you are. Try to do fun things together. The break will be good for all of you!

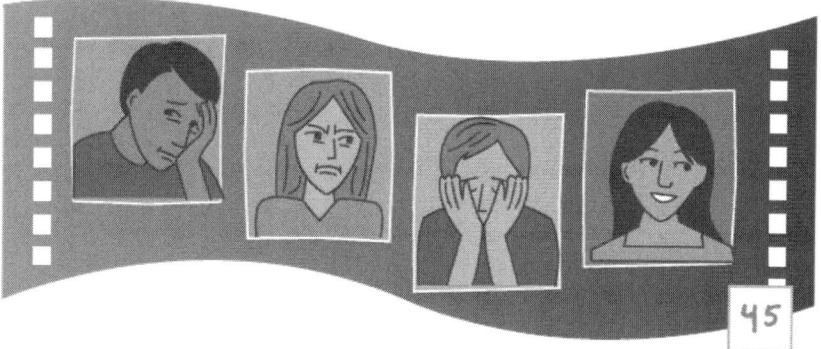

Dealing with hurtful remarks

Unfortunately, some kids may say mean things. Others speak before they think and before they get the facts. No matter the reason, it can hurt when kids make jokes or say hurtful things about you, cancer, or your parent.

What can you do?

→ Ignore the comment.

→ Say, "Hey, my dad has cancer. It's not funny. How would you feel if it was your dad?"

→ Being bullied? If standing up for yourself and saying "that's enough" doesn't work—talk with someone. Go to your parent, teacher, principal, or school counselor. You deserve to be treated with respect.

Do not protect yourself by a fence,
but rather by your friends.

—Czech proverb

Chapter 9

How you can help your parent

Here are some things that others have done to help their parent at home. Pick one or two things to try each week.

Help with care

Spend time with your parent.

Watch a movie together. Read the paper to your parent. Ask for help with your homework. Give hugs. Say, "I love you." Or just hang out in silence.

"Some days I felt really good about the little things I could do for my mom. Other times there wasn't anything I could do except just be with her. We didn't always have to talk. Even when I was quiet, I think my mom could sense my love." —Vanessa, age 16

Lend a hand.

Bring water or offer to make a snack or small meal.

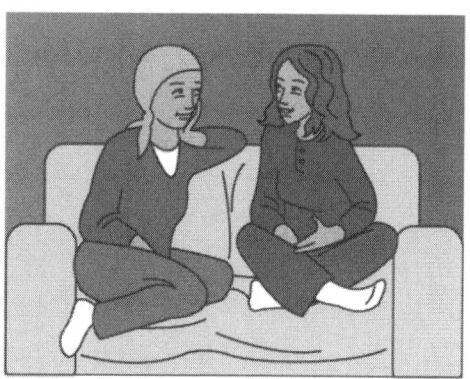

Help by being thoughtful

Try to be upbeat, but be "real," too.
Being positive can be good for you and your whole family. But
don't feel like you always have to act cheerful, especially if it's
not how you really feel. It's okay to share your thoughts with your
parent—and let them comfort you. Be yourself.

Be patient.
You are all under stress. If you find you are losing your cool, listen
to music, read, or go outside to shoot hoops or go for a run.

Share a laugh.
You've probably heard that laughter is good medicine. Watch a
comedy on TV with your parent or tell jokes if that's your thing.
Also, remember that you're not responsible for making everyone
happy. You can only do so much.

Buy your parent a new scarf or hat.
Your parent might enjoy a new hat or scarf if he or she has lost
their hair during treatment.

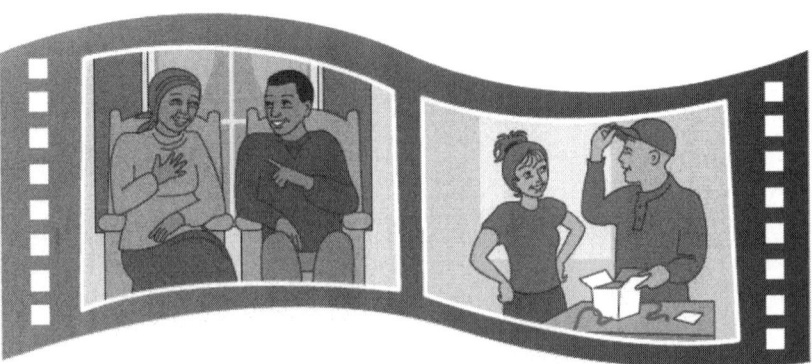

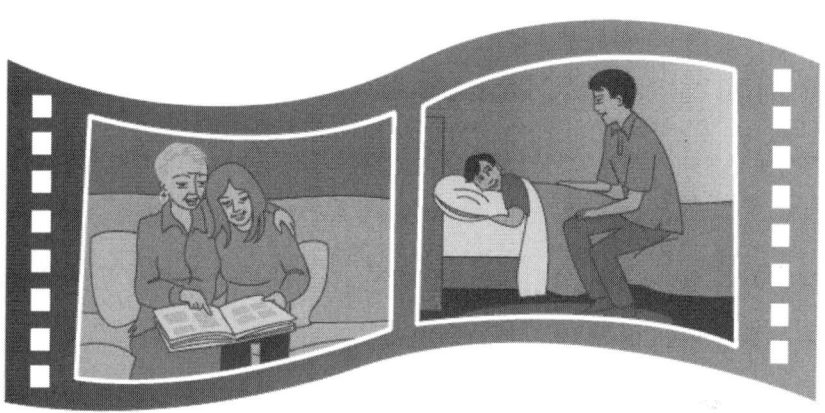

Help by staying involved

Keep your parent in the loop.
Tell your parent what you did today. Try to share what is going on in your life. Ask your parent how his or her day was.

Talk about family history.
Ask your parent about the past. Look through pictures or photo albums. Talk about what you're both most proud of, your best memories, and how you both have met challenges. Write, or make drawings, about what you and your parent share with each other.

Keep a journal together.
Write thoughts or poems, draw, or put photos in a notebook that the two of you share. This can help you share your feelings when it might be hard to speak them aloud.

Help with younger brothers and sisters.
Play with your brothers and sisters to give your parent a break. Pull out games or read a book with your siblings. This will help you stay close and also give your parent time to rest.

"Before my dad got cancer, I didn't take time to really notice all the stuff I had going for me. But I've learned to open my eyes more. Bad things happen in this world—like my dad getting cancer—but it's a pretty wonderful place, too. Even while there's been a lot of added pressure on our family, I've learned to appreciate every day more."
—Kenyatta, age 18

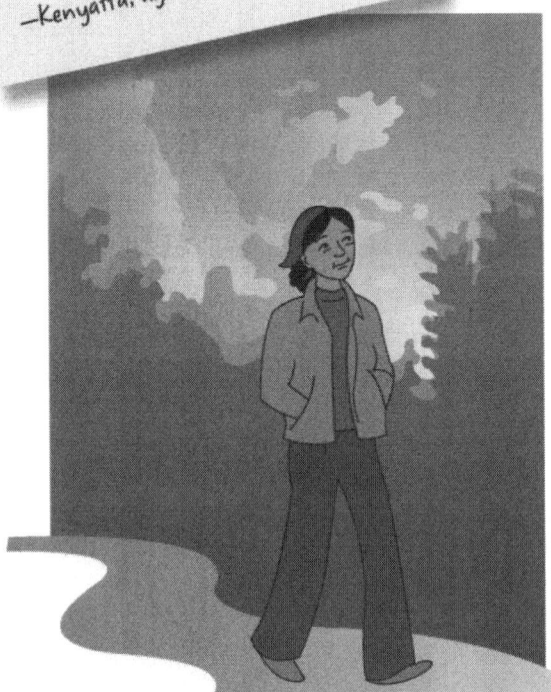

Chapter 10

After treatment

When your parent is finally done with treatment, you may feel a whole range of emotions. Part of you is glad it is over. Another part of you may miss the freedom or new responsibilities you had while your parent was getting treatment. You may feel confused that your parent still looks sick and is weaker than you expected. You may be afraid the cancer will come back. You may look at life differently now. All these feelings are normal. If you and your family are still feeling that life after treatment is harder than you thought it might be, you might want to talk to a counselor to get guidance through this time.

Things may not go back to exactly how they were before cancer came into your lives. Getting back to your "old life" may take a long time—or it may not happen as you expect.

Here are some things that others have to say about life after treatment. Do any of these kids sound like you?

Caleb talks about the "new normal":

"Now that my mom is done with chemo and radiation, things are pretty different. My older brother drove her to treatment. It was my job to get dinner and help my little sister, Jada, with homework each night. Now that Mom is better, Jada doesn't need as much help from me. For a while I was her hero. Look, I am glad Mom's treatment went well, but getting used to her being up and about is, well, different. My mom says it will take time." —Caleb, age 15

Sarah appreciates life more:

"I have to admit it, before my mom got sick we fought a lot—over what I was wearing, who I hung out with, or why I wasn't nicer to my little sister. After my mother got cancer, we pulled together more. My sister and I got tight. She looked up to me to make sure we were going to be all right. Now stuff like painting my nails or wearing cool clothes don't matter as much. I even help run a support group for kids at my school who have a sick parent." —Sarah, age 17

Jake is glad to have his dad back home:

"All I can say is that I never saw my dad cry until he finished his last chemo treatment. The doctors said they think they got all the cancer. My father was so emotional—glad to be alive. Then my mom and brother lost it, too. I have to say that I'm so glad my dad is better. I used to take him for granted. No more."
—Jake, age 16

Our greatest glory is

not in never failing,

but in rising up every time we fail.

—Ralph Waldo Emerson

What if treatment doesn't help?

If treatment doesn't help your parent, you and your family will face even more challenges. Hearing that your parent might die is very difficult. You may feel many of the same emotions you felt when you first learned that your mom or dad had cancer.

No booklet can give you all the answers or tell you exactly how you will feel. But when the future is so uncertain, teens say it helps to:

➡ **Make the most of the time you have.**
Do special things as a family. At home, make time for your mom or dad. Call and visit as much as you can if your parent is in the hospital. Write notes and draw pictures. Say "I love you" often.

If possible, try to have some special times together. If you have not gotten along in the past, you may want to let your parent know you love him or her.

➡ **Stay on track.**
When people get bad news, they often feel like they're living outside of themselves—that life is moving along without them. That's why it's important to keep a schedule. Get up at the same time each day. Go to school. Meet with friends.

➡ **Get help when you feel alone.**
Make sure you find people who can help you. In addition to your family, it may help to talk to a social worker, counselor, or people in a support group.

The past cannot be changed;

Cancer organizations can also help you during this very difficult time in your life. In Chapter 12, you'll find some organizations to contact.

"It was very hard to hear that my mom's treatment wasn't working anymore. She and I decided to make the most of each day. Some days we talk nonstop. Other times we just sit together and hold hands. But every day, I tell my mom how much I love her. You can't be afraid to love. Not ever. I learned that."

—Emily, age 16

the future is still in your power. —Hugh White

If your parent passes away, know that...

You'll always have memories.
Your parent will always be part of your life. Hold on to your memories of the good times. Don't feel guilty that you're not respecting your parent's memory when you think about something funny that your parent did or said. By laughing and smiling you are bringing back just a little of what was so special about your parent.

The pain will get less intense with time.
At first the pain may be so strong that you might wonder whether you will ever feel happy again. Time has a way of healing. Not being sad every day doesn't mean that you have forgotten your parent. It just means that you are starting to heal.

Everyone grieves in his or her own way.
Some teens grieve for their parent's death by crying. Others get quiet and spend time by themselves. Some find that they need to be around friends and talk. Others get very angry. In any case, most people find it helps to keep a regular routine. There is no right way or wrong way to grieve. It's okay to deal with loss at your own pace.

Your parent would want you to be happy.
Stay open to new experiences. Write about your thoughts. Make small changes that give your life new meaning.

Life will change.
Life won't be the same as before, but it can be rich and full again. Keep believing this.

Chapter 11

The road ahead

It can be hard to stay calm when you aren't sure what the future holds. You may be thinking—will my parent survive cancer? Will the cancer come back? Will life ever be the same? Will I laugh again?

While no one can know the future, there are things you can do to make your life a little more stable:

Keep talking and pulling together as a family. You may find that cancer has drawn you closer together and made you appreciate each other more than ever.

Discover your own needs. Don't let others tell you how you should feel. Allow yourself to cope at your own pace and in your own way.

Remember that you're growing as a person. Many teens say that having a parent with cancer has made them more sympathetic, more responsible, and stronger.

"Don't get me wrong, I'm so glad that treatment is over. Seeing my stepdad so sick was hard to take. But now that he's back home, well, bedtime is back to 10:00, no more late night TV, I have to say where I'll be and when I'll be home... basically, we're back to the old rules." —Monica, age 17

57

Accept people's help. Right now you may feel lonelier than you ever have in your life. But you are not alone. Family, friends, support groups, neighbors, and counselors are there to lend a helping hand, listen to you, and be there for you.

Appreciate each day. Many teens who have a parent with cancer say that they learned to see the world more clearly. In time you may come to appreciate things you may have overlooked in the past.

Maybe you have noticed that little things seem to have more meaning for you these days. Take some time to write these thoughts down, even if they seem small:

No booklet or person can tell you exactly how everything is going to work out. Cancer is tough, and your life may never be quite the same. But in the end, you will get through it. Why? You're strong. And you are capable—even if you don't always feel that way.

To know the road ahead, ask those coming back.

—Chinese proverb

Chapter 12

Learning more on your own

It's great that you want to learn more. Keep in mind that cancer treatments are getting better all the time. Make sure that what you read or see is up to date and accurate. Talk with your parent or other trusted adult about what you find. Share the articles or books you've found with them. Ask them any questions you may have. You can get information from:

➡ **Your school or public library**
Ask the librarian to help you find the information or support that you're looking for in books, magazines, videos, or on the Internet.

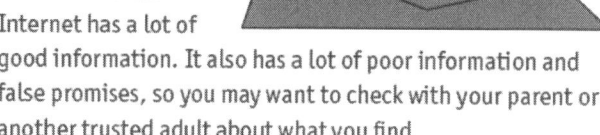

➡ **The Internet**
Use an Internet search engine and type in general words like "parent" and "cancer" together to get started. Keep in mind that the Internet has a lot of good information. It also has a lot of poor information and false promises, so you may want to check with your parent or another trusted adult about what you find.

➡ **Your parent's hospital or clinic**
Visit the patient education office at your parent's hospital, if there is one. Or, ask if you can go with your parent during their visit to the doctor—to learn more.

Help is a phone call or web site away

Here are some places to contact for help. You can call them or visit their Web site for more information.

National Cancer Institute (NCI)

NCI has up-to-date, accurate information for you and your family. Get answers to your questions and learn more by calling us, visiting our Web site, or ordering our publications. We provide information in both English and Spanish on types of cancer, treatment, clinical trials, supportive care, complementary and alternative medicine, as well as on screening, prevention, and genetics. You will also find a dictionary of cancer terms, and a drug dictionary, on our site. We are a federal government agency that is part of the U.S. Department of Health and Human Services.

Find more organizations:

Visit **www.cancer.gov** and type "national organizations" into the search box. You will find a list of *National Organizations That Offer Cancer-Related Services*. These organizations provide emotional, financial, and/or informational support to people with cancer and their families. Or call 1-800-4-CANCER (1-800-422-6237) to learn more.

Web..................... www.cancer.gov and
www.cancer.gov/espanol

Online Chat .... www.cancer.gov/livehelp

E-mail .... cancergovstaff@mail.nih.gov

Phone.................. 1-800-4-CANCER (1-800-422-6237)

Publications .... www.cancer.gov/publications or call
1-800-4-CANCER

American Cancer Society (ACS)

ACS is a nationwide, community-based voluntary health organization. ACS offers a variety of services and programs for patients and their families. ACS also supports research, provides printed materials, and conducts educational programs. Staff can accept calls and distribute publications in Spanish.

Web..................... **www.cancer.org**

Phone.................. 1-800-ACS-2345 (1-800-227-2345)

TTY...................... 1-866-228-4327

American Society of Clinical Oncology (ASCO)

ASCO has oncologist-approved cancer information to help patients and families make informed health care decisions. ASCO's site also has podcasts and videos for patients and family members. The site also includes a section on camps and retreats for families and children touched by cancer.

Web..................... **www.cancer.net**

Cancer Support Community (CSC)

The Cancer Support Community (CSC) was formed by the merger of Gilda's Club Worldwide and The Wellness Community. CSC is an international non-profit organization that has a network of personalized services and education for all people affected by cancer. Its free programs include support groups, counseling, education, and healthy lifestyle initiatives. These support services are available online and through local affiliates.

Web..................... **www.cancersupportcommunity.org**

E-mail .... help@cancersupportcommunity.org

Phone.................. 1-888-793-WELL (1-888-793-9355)

CancerCare

CancerCare provides free professional support services and publications to anyone affected by cancer, including the patient's children and loved ones. Services include counseling and support groups, education, financial assistance, and practical help. CancerCare also accepts calls and distributes publications in Spanish. Limited grants are available to eligible families for cancer-related costs like transportation and childcare.

Web...................... **www.cancercare.org**

E-mail .... info@cancercare.org

Phone.................. 1-800-813-HOPE (1-800-813-4673)

Chart A: Cancer team members

TEAM MEMBER	WHAT THEY DO
Nurse	A health professional trained to care for people who are ill or disabled
Nutritionist/ dietitian	A health professional with special training in nutrition who can help with dietary choices
Oncologist	A doctor who specializes in treating people with cancer. Some oncologists specialize in certain types of cancer or certain types of cancer treatment.
Patient educator	Educates patients and families about illness
Pharmacist	Dispenses medicines for patients
Physical therapist	Teaches exercises and physical activities that help patients gain more muscle strength and movement
Psychiatrist	A doctor who treats mental health problems, including depression, with medicine and talk therapy
Psychologist	Talks with patients and their families about emotional and personal matters and helps them make decisions
Radiologist	A doctor who looks at x-rays and other images of the body
Religious or spiritual leader	Addresses the spiritual and emotional health of patients and their families. This can be a chaplain, minister, priest, rabbi, imam, or youth group leader.
Social worker	Talks with people and their families about emotional or physical needs and helps them find support services
Surgeon	A doctor who removes or repairs a part of the body by operating on the patient

Chart B: Monitoring Tests

TEST	PURPOSE
Biopsy	Used to find out whether a tumor or abnormality is cancer. Benign means it is not cancer. Malignant means that it is cancer.
Blood test	Checks the blood to see whether the balance of the cells and chemicals is normal
Bone marrow aspiration	Collects a small sample of cells from inside a bone to be examined under a microscope
CAT scan or CT scan (Computerized axial tomography)	Uses **x-rays** and a computer to produce three-dimensional (3-D) images of the inside of the body
MRI (Magnetic resonance imaging)	Uses radio and magnetic waves to make images of organs and other tissues inside the body
PET scan (Positron emission tomography)	Uses computerized pictures of areas inside the body to find cancer cells
Spinal tap (Lumbar puncture)	Collects a sample of the fluid inside the spine to be examined under a microscope
Ultrasound (Ultrasonography)	Uses high-frequency sound waves to make images of organs and tissues inside the body
X-ray	Takes a picture of the inside of the body using high-energy radiation

PROCEDURE (What happens)
A doctor removes a sample of tissue in one of two ways: with a long needle (needle biopsy) or by making a small cut (surgical biopsy).
A nurse or technician inserts a needle into a vein, usually in the arm. Then he or she draws blood.
A needle is used to remove a small sample of tissue from a bone (usually the hip bone).
The patient lies flat on a table, which moves through a large tube while a series of x-rays is taken.
The patient lies flat on a table, which moves through a large tube while an MRI machine scans the body for several minutes.
The patient gets an injection of a special dye and then a machine takes computerized pictures of areas inside the body.
A needle is used to remove fluid from the spine in the lower back.
A technician moves a small handheld device over an area on the patient's body. An image appears on the computer screen.
The patient is placed in front of the x-ray machine or lies on a table.

Glossary

What the Terms Mean

This list can help you learn some words that your parents or the doctors and nurses may use. Don't be afraid to ask questions when you don't understand what they are talking about. These people are there to help you, too.

Benign: Not cancer. Benign tumors do not spread to the tissues around them or to other parts of the body.

Biological therapy: Treatment to help the body's immune system fight infections, cancer, and other diseases. It is also used to reduce certain side effects of cancer treatment. Other names include immunotherapy, biotherapy, or BRM (biological response modifier) therapy.

Bone marrow: The soft, sponge-like tissue in the center of most bones. It makes white blood cells, red blood cells, and platelets.

Cancer: A term for diseases in which abnormal cells divide without control. Cancer cells can invade nearby tissues and can spread through the bloodstream and lymphatic system to other parts of the body. These are the main types of cancer:

- **Carcinoma** starts in the skin or in tissues that line or cover internal organs.
- **Central nervous system cancers** begin in the tissues of the brain and spinal cord.
- **Leukemia** starts in blood-forming tissue such as the bone marrow. Large numbers of abnormal blood cells form and enter the bloodstream.
- **Lymphoma** and **multiple myeloma** begin in the cells of the immune system.
- **Sarcoma** starts in bone, cartilage, fat, muscle, blood vessels, or other connective or supportive tissue.

Cell: The individual unit that makes up the tissues of the body. All living things are made up of one or more cells.

Chemotherapy: Treatment with medicines that destroy cancer cells. Also called chemo. Chemo is most often given intravenously (IV) (through a blood vessel). Some chemo can also be taken as a pill.

Depression: A mental condition marked by ongoing feelings of sadness, despair, loss of energy, and difficulty dealing with normal daily life. Other symptoms of depression include feeling worthless or hopeless, loss of pleasure in activities, changes in eating or sleeping habits, and thoughts of death or suicide. Depression can affect anyone, and can be successfully treated.

Diagnosis: The process of identifying a disease, such as cancer, from its signs and symptoms.

Hormone: A chemical made by glands in your body. Hormones move in the bloodstream. They control the actions of certain cells or organs. Some hormones can also be made in the laboratory.

Hormone therapy: Treatment that adds, blocks, or removes hormones. To slow or stop the growth of certain cancers (such as prostate and breast cancer), synthetic hormones or other drugs may be given to block the body's natural hormones.

Immune system: Organs and cells that defend the body against infections and other diseases.

Inherited: Transmitted through genes that have been passed from parents to their offspring (children).

Intravenous: Into or within a vein. Intravenous usually refers to a way of giving a drug or other substance through a needle or tube inserted into a vein. Also called IV.

IV: Into or within a vein. IV usually refers to a way of giving a drug or other substance through a needle or tube inserted into a vein. Also called intravenous.

Leukemia: Cancer that starts in blood-forming tissue such as the bone marrow and causes large numbers of blood cells to form and enter the bloodstream.

Malignant: Cancer. Malignant tumors can invade nearby tissue and spread to other parts of the body.

Metastasis: The spread of cancer from one part of the body to another. A tumor formed by cells that have spread is called a metastatic tumor or a metastasis. The metastatic tumor contains cells that are like those in the original (primary) tumor.

Radiation therapy: The use of high-energy radiation from x-rays, gamma rays, neutrons, protons, and other sources to destroy cancer cells and shrink tumors. Radiation may come from a machine outside the body (external-beam radiation therapy), or it may come from radioactive material placed in the body near cancer cells (internal radiation therapy).

Recurrence: Cancer that has recurred (come back), usually after a period of time during which the cancer could not be detected. The cancer may come back to the same place as the original (primary) tumor or to another place in the body. Also called recurrent cancer.

Relapse: The return of cancer after a period of improvement.

Remission: A decrease in or disappearance of signs and symptoms of cancer. In partial remission, some, but not all, signs and symptoms of cancer have disappeared. In complete remission, all signs and symptoms of cancer have disappeared, although cancer still may be in the body.

Risk factor: Something that increases the chance of developing a disease. Some examples of risk factors for cancer are age, a family history of certain cancers, use of tobacco products, being exposed to radiation or certain chemicals, infection with certain viruses or bacteria, and certain genetic changes.

Side effect: A problem that occurs when treatment affects healthy tissues or organs. Some common side effects of cancer treatment are fatigue, pain, nausea, vomiting, decreased blood cell counts, hair loss, and mouth sores.

Stem cell: A cell from which other types of cells develop. For example, blood cells develop from blood-forming stem cells.

Stem cell transplant: A method of replacing immature blood-forming cells in the bone marrow that have been destroyed by drugs, radiation, or disease. Stem cells are injected into the patient and make healthy blood cells. A stem cell transplant may be autologous (using a patient's own stem cells that were saved before treatment), allogeneic (using stem cells donated by someone who is not an identical twin), or syngeneic (using stem cells donated by an identical twin).

Support group: A group of people with similar concerns who help each other by sharing experiences, knowledge, and information.

Surgery: A procedure to remove or repair a part of the body or to find out whether disease is present. An operation.

Tissue: A group or layer of cells that work together to perform a specific function.

Tumor: An abnormal mass of tissue that results when cells divide more than they should or do not die when they should. Tumors may be benign (not cancer), or malignant (cancer). Also called neoplasm.

Printed in Great Britain
by Amazon